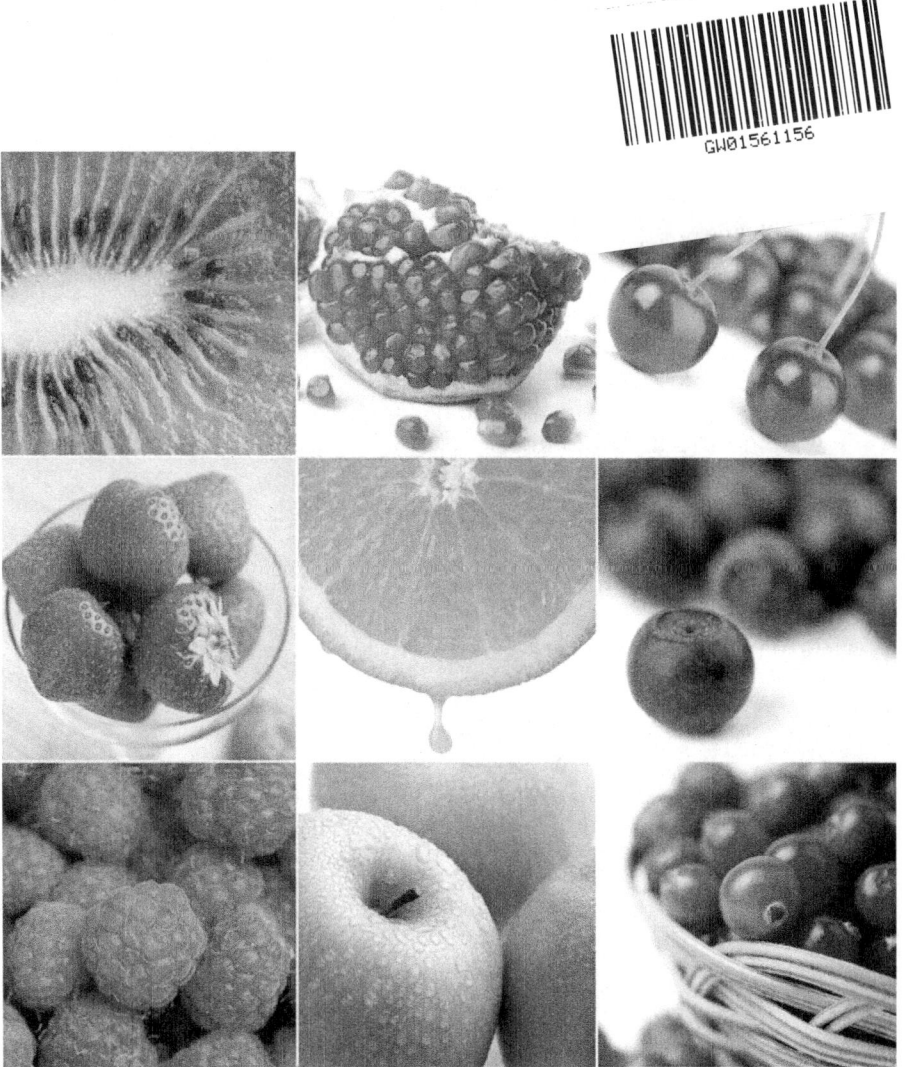

Alkaline and Acidic
Food Chart Report

Alkaline and Acidic Food Chart Report

Table of Contents

Getting More Alkaline Into Your Diet 4

Alkaline Diet and Health 12

Alkaline Diet and Back Pain 13

Alkalinity and Chemotheraphy 14

Alkaline Diet and Growth Hormone 14

Alkaline Diet and Muscle Mass 15

Alkaline Diet 16

What is PRAL: Potential Renal Acid Load? 17

Alkaline Diet Research 19

Alkaline Vegetables 20

Low Acid Diet 32

    Tired of Feeling the Burn? Low-Acid Diet May Help 32

Alkaline Diet Research 34

Fruits Low in Acidity 34

Alkaline and Acidic Food Chart Report

Getting More Alkaline Into Your Diet

The pH miracle diet is a revolutionary new way to look at how you eat. The essentials of the diet are to keep the ph balance of food intake at 80% alkaline with 20% acidity. The goal with this diet is to match the ph level of the bloodstream, which runs on the alkaline side. This task can be daunting for many because foods that most people love to indulge themselves on are considered high in acidity. The goal in adding more alkaline into your diet is to identify good sources of alkaline. Creating a comprehensive list of alkaline producing foods will help you make the most of the pH miracle diet.

Alkalizing foods have a tonic effect on the body. By neutralizing the acidity in the bloodstream, alkaline foods act as a breath of fresh air to the system regenerating and restoring damaged cells. Diets high in acidic foods cause the body to break down prematurely, the bloodstream carries these acid bombs throughout the system wreaking havoc in their

Alkaline and Acidic Food Chart Report

wake. By determining what foods have an alkalizing effect on the body, we can incorporate them into our diet in larger amounts, setting the pH levels in the bloodstream to the optimum level. On average, the pH level of human blood is between 7.35 and 7.45; levels 7 and above are considered alkaline.

Vegetables and fruits are the easiest ways to get more alkaline into your diet.

Vegetables that are alkalizing are: alfalfa, barley grass, beets, beet greens, broccoli, cabbage, carrot, cauliflower, celery, chard greens, collard greens, cucumber, dandelions, eggplant, garlic, green beans, green peas, kale, kohlrabi, lettuce, mushrooms, mustard greens, nightshade veggies, onions, parsnips, peas, peppers, pumpkin, radishes, rutabaga, sea veggies, spinach, sprouts, sweet potatoes, tomatoes, watercress, wheat grass, and wild greens.

Fruits that have an alkalizing effect are: apples, apricots, avocados, bananas, berries, blackberries,

Alkaline and Acidic Food Chart Report

cantaloupe, cherries, coconut, currants, dates, figs, grapes, grapefruit, honeydew, lemons, limes, muskmelons, nectarines, oranges, peaches, pears, pineapple, raisins, raspberries, rhubarb, strawberries, tangerines, tomatoes, tropical fruits, and watermelon. Also, since cherry juice is alkaline, it will help to maintain your pH balance to healthy alkaline levels. Visit www.TraverseBayFarms.com to learn more about tart cherry juice.

Protein can be a problem when attempting to add more alkaline into your diet. All protein derived from animals is acidic. It is possible to add protein to your diet that will have an alkalizing effect in your bloodstream. Proteins that are alkaline are: almonds, chestnuts, millet, tempeh, tofu, and whey protein powder.

Food is nothing without the spices, herbs and sweeteners that give it that extra bit of character. You can add these alkalizing additions to your culinary efforts to bring your PH levels into balance. Alkalizing

Alkaline and Acidic Food Chart Report

condiments are: cinnamon, curry, ginger, mustard, chili pepper, sea salt, stevia, miso, tamari, and all herbs.

Minerals are essential to optimum health. Paying attention to which minerals have alkalizing effects can add the proper balance to your blood pH. Minerals that have an alkalizing effect on the body are: cesium, potassium, sodium, calcium, and magnesium.

There are other incidentals that can make adding alkaline to your diet even easier. Other ways to add alkaline to your diet are: apple cider vinegar, alkaline antioxidant water, bee pollen, lecithin granules, molasses, probiotic cultures, soured dairy products, green juices, veggie juices, fresh fruit juice, and mineral water.

Knowing which foods and supplements that add alkaline to your pH levels is just the beginning. Implementing them is the next step which takes planning and commitment. After adding these healing

Alkaline and Acidic Food Chart Report

foods to your diet you can test your bodys pH levels with a saliva strip test available at most health food stores. Keeping your pH level between 7 and 8 is the target for good health.

Remember the goal of the pH miracle diet is to have the alkaline intake higher than your acidic intake. This does not mean that you can't enjoy the foods that are higher in acidity, quite the contrary; the balance of your diet should be geared toward alkaline producing foods. By maintaining a proper pH balance you can ensure that your body is performing at its optimum level.

Alkaline and Acidic Food Chart Report

How To Determine Your Body pH Balance

Herbal programs may work more effectively when the pH is in balance. Get more from your supplementation program by balancing your pH. Your body is able to assimilate minerals and nutrients properly only when its pH is balanced. It is therefore possible for you to be taking healthy nutrients and yet be unable to absorb or use them. If you are not getting the results you expected from your nutritional or herbal program, look for an acid alkaline imbalance. Even the right herbal program may not work if your body's pH is out of balance. Check out www.OrchardOfHealth.com (Orchard of Health) to learn more about pH balances and food.

Note that a food's acid or alkaline-forming tendency in the body has nothing to do with the actual pH of the food itself. For example, lemons are very acidic, however the end-products they produce after digestion and assimilation are very alkaline so lemons are alkaline-forming in the body.

Alkaline and Acidic Food Chart Report

Likewise, meat will test alkaline before digestion but it leaves very acidic residue in the body so, like nearly all animal products, meat is very acid-forming.

The correct ratio of acid and alkaline forming foods is difficult to know since the balance is altered by chewing, food preparation, individual lifestyle, genetics, exercise, and mental outlook. However, those prone to infections, viruses, excess mucus problems and other toxic acidic conditions need to increase their alkaline diet.

The Saliva PH test is a simple test you can do to measure your susceptibility to cancer, heart disease, osteoporosis, arthritis, and many other degenerative diseases.

There is a simple way of measuring saliva pH. First, you must wait at least 2 hours after eating. Fill your mouth with saliva and then swallow it. Repeat this step to help ensure that your saliva is clean. Then the third time, put some of your saliva onto the pH paper.

Alkaline and Acidic Food Chart Report

The pH paper should turn blue. This indicates that your saliva is slightly alkaline at a healthy pH of 7.4. If it is not blue, compare the color with the chart that comes with the pH paper. If your saliva is acid (below pH of 7.0) wait two hours and repeat the test.

Some health food stores and pharmacies stock pH paper. What you are looking for is narrow range pH paper measuring pH 4.5 to 7.5 or pH 4.5 to 8.5. These pH strips to measure acid/alkaline balance pH belong in every family medicine kit, right beside the thermometer to measure body temperature.

pH paper for the test are relatively easy to acquire. Some health food stores and pharmacies stock pH paper. What you are looking for is narrow range pH paper measuring pH 4.5 to 7.5 or pH 4.5 to 8.5. These pH strips to measure acid/alkaline balance belong in every family medicine kit, right beside the thermometer to measure body temperature.

Alkaline and Acidic Food Chart Report

Alkaline Diet and Health

Alkaline diets result in a more alkaline urine pH and may result in reduced calcium in the urine, however, this may not reflect total calcium balance because of other buffers such as phosphate. There is no substantial evidence that this improves bone health or protects from osteoporosis. However, alkaline diets may result in a number of health benefits as outlined below. The website www.DiscountDietSite.com Discount Diet Site offers additional research and information about diet and health.

Increased fruits and vegetables in an alkaline diet would improve the potassium / sodium ratio and may benefit bone health, reduce muscle wasting, as well as mitigate other chronic diseases such as hypertension and strokes.

The resultant increase in growth hormone with an alkaline diet may improve many outcomes from cardiovascular health to memory and cognition.

Alkaline and Acidic Food Chart Report

An increase in intracellular magnesium, which is required for the function of many enzyme systems, is another added benefit of the alkaline diet. Available magnesium, which is required to activate vitamin D, would result in numerous added benefits in the vitamin D apocrine/exocrine systems.

Alkalinity may result in added benefit for some chemotherapeutic agents that require a higher pH.

From the evidence outlined above, it would be prudent to consider an alkaline diet to reduce morbidity and mortality of chronic disease that are plaguing our aging population. One of the first considerations in an alkaline diet, which includes more fruits and vegetables, is to know what type of soil they were grown in since this may significantly influence the mineral content.

Alkaline Diet and Back Pain

There is some evidence that chronic low back pain improves with the supplementation of alkaline minerals. With supplementation there was a slight but

Alkaline and Acidic Food Chart Report

significant Increase in blood pH and intracellular magnesium. Ensuring that there is enough intracellular magnesium allows for the proper function of enzyme systems and also allows for activation of vitamin D. This in turn has been shown to improve back pain.

Alkalinity and Chemotheraphy

The effectiveness of chemotherapeutic agents is markedly influenced by pH. Numerous agents such as epirubicin and adriamycin require an alkaline media to be more effective. Others, such as cisplatin, mitomycin C, and thiotepa, are more cytotoxic in an acid media. However, there is no scientific literature establishing the benefit of an alkaline diet for the prevention of cancer at this time.

Alkaline Diet and Growth Hormone

It has long been known that severe forms of metabolic acidosis in children, such as renal tubular acidosis, are associated with low levels of growth hormone with resultant short stature. Correction of

Alkaline and Acidic Food Chart Report

the acidosis with bicarbonate or potassium citrate increases growth hormone significantly and improved growth. The use of enough potassium bicarbonate in the diet to neutralize the daily net acid load in postmenopausal women resulted in a significant increase in growth hormone and resultant osteocalcin. Improving growth hormone levels may improve quality of life, reduce cardiovascular risk factors, improve body composition, and even improve memory and cognition.

Alkaline Diet and Muscle Mass

As we age, there is a loss of muscle mass, which may predispose to falls and fractures. A three-year study looking at a diet rich in potassium, such as fruits and vegetables, as well as a reduced acid load, resulted in preservation of muscle mass in older men and women. Conditions such as chronic renal failure that result in chronic metabolic acidosis result in accelerated breakdown in skeletal muscle. Correction of acidosis may preserve muscle mass in conditions where muscle wasting is common such as diabetic

Alkaline and Acidic Food Chart Report

ketosis, trauma, sepsis, chronic obstructive lung disease, and renal failure.

Alkaline Diet

When it comes to the pH and net acid load in the human diet, there has been considerable change from the hunter gather civilization to the present. With industrialization, there has been an decrease in potassium (K) compared to sodium (Na) and an increase in chloride compared to bicarbonate found in the diet. The ratio of potassium to sodium has reversed, K/Na previously was 10 to 1 whereas the modern diet has a ratio of 1 to 3. It is generally accepted that agricultural humans today have a diet poor in magnesium and potassium as well as fiber and rich in saturated fat, simple sugars, sodium, and chloride as compared to the preagricultural period.

This results in a diet that may induce metabolic acidosis which is mismatched to the genetically determined nutritional requirements. With aging, there is a gradual loss of renal acid-base regulatory

Alkaline and Acidic Food Chart Report

function and a resultant increase in diet-induced metabolic acidosis while on the modern diet. A low-carb high-protein diet with its increased acid load results in many changes in urinary chemistry. Urinary magnesium levels, urinary citrate and pH are decreased, urinary calcium, undissociated uric acid, and phosphate are increased. All of these result in an increased risk for kidney stones.

As we age, there is a loss of muscle mass, which may predispose to falls and fractures. A three-year study looking at a diet rich in potassium, such as fruits and vegetables, as well as a reduced acid load, resulted in preservation of muscle mass in older men and women. There is also some evidence that chronic low back pain improves with the supplementation of alkaline minerals.

What is PRAL: Potential Renal Acid Load?

PRAL value is calculated from a formula developed to assess the acidity of foods and diets.

Alkaline and Acidic Food Chart Report

PRAL formula:

PRAL = 0.49 x protein + 0.037 x phosphorus - 0.021 x potassium - 0.026 x magnesium - 0.013 x calcium

Today, there is a general consensus that diet can markedly affect acid-base status and that a person's acid load can be specifically manipulated by dietary means. An established method of estimating acid loads of foods or diets is by calculating the potential renal acid load (PRAL). PRAL provides an estimate of the production of endogenous acid that exceeds the level of alkali produced for given amounts of foods ingested daily. The concept of PRAL calculation is physiologically based and takes into account different intestinal absorption rates of individual minerals and of sulfurcontaining protein, as well as the amount of sulfate produced from metabolized proteins. This method of calculation was experimentally validated in healthy adults, and it showed that, under controlled conditions, acid loads and renal net acid excretion (NAE) can be reliably estimated from diet composition.

Alkaline and Acidic Food Chart Report

Alkaline Diet Research

Muscle mass gradually declines after age 50, and muscle loss leads to muscle weakness; greater risks of falls, fractures, and disability; and loss of independence. There is plausible evidence that the composition of diets with respect to acid-base balance is a contributing factor.

Protein and cereal grains are metabolized to acidic residues, and fruit and vegetables are metabolized to alkaline residues. In general, American diets are acidic, generating 75–100 mEq acid/d. With the decline in renal function that occurs with aging, older persons are not able to excrete the excess hydrogen ions, and they develop mild but slowly increasing metabolic acidosis. Metabolic acidosis has been linked to muscle wasting in chronic renal failure and in obese subjects who were acidotic while following weight-loss diets; correction of the acidosis has been shown to reverse the muscle wasting in these 2 conditions.

Alkaline and Acidic Food Chart Report

Alkaline Vegetables

List of high-alkaline vegetables based on PRAL values.

Low-Acid Vegetables	PRAL value
Parsley, freeze-dried	-109
Radishes, oriental, dried	-75
Chives, freeze-dried	-60
Tomatoes, sun-dried	-58
Peppers, sweet, green, freeze-dried	-52
Peppers, sweet, red, freeze-dried	-52
Seaweed, agar, dried	-47
Carrot, dehydrated	-42
Peppers, ancho, dried	-41
Leeks, (bulb and lower-leaf portion), freeze-dried	-39
Peppers, pasilla, dried	-35
Peppers, hot chile, sun-dried	-31

Alkaline and Acidic Food Chart Report

Tomato powder	-30
Kanpyo, (dried gourd strips)	-29
Tomatoes, sun-dried, packed in oil, drained	-28
Potatoes, mashed, dehydrated, granules with milk, dry form	-28
Onions, dehydrated flakes	-24
Shallots, freeze-dried	-23
Mushrooms, shiitake, dried	-20
Beet greens, cooked, boiled, drained, without salt	-20
Beet greens, cooked, boiled, drained, with salt	-20
Tomato products, canned, paste, with salt added	-18
Tomato products, canned, paste, without salt added	-18
Epazote, raw	-17
Beet greens, raw	-17
Butterbur, (fuki), raw	-15
Potatoes, mashed, dehydrated, flakes without	-15

Alkaline and Acidic Food Chart Report

milk, dry form

Yam, raw   -15

Potato flour   -14

Low-Acid Vegetables	PRAL value
Amaranth leaves, cooked, boiled, drained, with salt	-14
Amaranth leaves, cooked, boiled, drained, without salt	-14
Fireweed, leaves, raw	-14
Amaranth leaves, raw	-14
Lemon grass (citronella), raw	-13
Taro, tahitian, raw	-13
Pepeao, dried	-13
Taro leaves, raw	-12
Chard, swiss, cooked, boiled, drained, with salt	-12
Spinach, raw	-12

Alkaline and Acidic Food Chart Report

Chard, swiss, cooked, boiled, drained, without salt	-12
Taro, tahitian, cooked, without salt	-12
Taro, tahitian, cooked, with salt	-12
Yam, cooked, boiled, drained, or baked, with salt	-12
Arrowhead, raw	-12
Yam, cooked, boiled, drained, or baked, without salt	-12
Jute, potherb, cooked, boiled, drained, with salt	-11
Purslane, cooked, boiled, drained, with salt	-11
Vinespinach, (basella), raw	-11
Purslane, raw	-11
Chrysanthemum, garland, cooked, boiled, drained, without salt	-11
Chrysanthemum, garland, raw	-11
Purslane, cooked, boiled, drained, without salt	-11
Balsam-pear (bitter gourd), leafy tips, cooked, boiled, drained, with salt	-11

Alkaline and Acidic Food Chart Report

Cress, garden, raw	-11
Kale, scotch, raw	-11
Balsam-pear (bitter gourd), leafy tips, cooked, boiled, drained, without salt	-11
Parsley, fresh	-11
Chrysanthemum leaves, raw	-11
Chrysanthemum, garland, cooked, boiled, drained, with salt	-11
Yautia (tannier), raw	-11

Low-Acid Vegetables	PRAL value
Jute, potherb, raw	-11
Jute, potherb, cooked, boiled, drained, without salt	-11
Potatoes, scalloped, dry mix, unprepared	-10
Mustard spinach, (tendergreen), raw	-10
Wasabi, root, raw	-10
Spinach, cooked, boiled, drained, with salt	-10

Alkaline and Acidic Food Chart Report

Arrowhead, cooked, boiled, drained, without salt	-10
Lambsquarters, raw	-10
Balsam-pear (bitter gourd), leafy tips, raw	-10
Potatoes, microwaved, cooked in skin, skin, without salt	-10
Waterchestnuts, chinese, (matai), raw	-10
Arrowhead, cooked, boiled, drained, with salt	-10
Bamboo shoots, cooked, boiled, drained, without salt	-10
Bamboo shoots, cooked, boiled, drained, with salt	-10
Borage, cooked, boiled, drained, with salt	-10
Borage, cooked, boiled, drained, without salt	-10
Spinach, cooked, boiled, drained, without salt	-10
Potatoes, microwaved, cooked, in skin, skin with salt	-10
Taro, raw	-10
Coriander (cilantro) leaves, raw	-10

Alkaline and Acidic Food Chart Report

Borage, raw	-10
Sweet potato leaves, cooked, steamed, with salt	-9
Taro leaves, cooked, steamed, without salt	-9
Sweet potato leaves, cooked, steamed, without salt	-9
Squash, winter, acorn, cooked, baked, without salt	-9
Taro, leaves, cooked, steamed, with salt	-9
Squash, winter, acorn, cooked, baked, with salt	-9
Potatoes, Russet, flesh and skin, baked	-9
Potatoes, hashed brown, home-prepared	-9
Cardoon, cooked, boiled, drained, with salt	-9
Gourd, dishcloth (towelgourd), cooked, boiled, drained, with salt	-9

Low-Acid Vegetables	PRAL value
Cowpeas (blackeyes), immature seeds, raw	-9

Alkaline and Acidic Food Chart Report

Fungi, Cloud ears, dried	-9
Cowpeas, leafy tips, raw	-9
Beans, pinto, immature seeds, frozen, unprepared	-9
Cardoon, cooked, boiled, drained, without salt	-9
Cardoon, raw	-9
Gourd, dishcloth (towelgourd), cooked, boiled, drained, without salt	-9
Potatoes, baked, skin, with salt	-8
Drumstick leaves, cooked, boiled, drained, with salt	-8
Spinach, canned, regular pack, drained solids	-8
Dandelion greens, raw	-8
Butterbur, cooked, boiled, drained, with salt	-8
Tomato products, canned, puree, without salt added	-8
Chard, swiss, raw	-8
Cornsalad, raw	-8
Potatoes, white, flesh and skin, baked	-8

Alkaline and Acidic Food Chart Report

Butterbur, cooked, boiled, drained, without salt	-8
Taro, cooked, without salt	-8
Arugula, raw	-8
Sweet potato leaves, raw	-8
Potatoes, baked, skin, without salt	-8
Cowpeas (blackeyes), immature seeds, cooked, boiled, drained, with salt	-8
Drumstick pods, cooked, boiled, drained, with salt	-8
Sweet potato, cooked, baked in skin, without salt	-8
Cowpeas (blackeyes), immature seeds, cooked, boiled, drained, without salt	-8
Potatoes, red, flesh and skin, baked	-8
Drumstick leaves, cooked, boiled, drained, without salt	-8
Potato, baked, flesh and skin, without salt	-8
Bamboo shoots, raw	-8
Mountain yam, hawaii, cooked, steamed, with salt	-8

Alkaline and Acidic Food Chart Report

Lotus root, raw	-8

Low-Acid Vegetables	PRAL value
Mountain yam, hawaii, raw	-8
Mountain yam, hawaii, cooked, steamed, without salt	-8
Kale, raw	-8
Tomato products, canned, puree, with salt added	-8
Chicory greens, raw	-8
Nopales, raw	-8
Mushrooms, Chanterelle, raw	-8
Dock, raw	-8
Drumstick pods, cooked, boiled, drained, without salt	-8
Ginger root, raw	-8
Taro, cooked, with salt	-8
Drumstick pods, raw	-8

Alkaline and Acidic Food Chart Report

Potatoes, baked, flesh and skin, with salt   -8

Sweet potato, cooked, baked in skin, with salt   -8

Alkaline and Acidic Food Chart Report

Alkaline and Acidic Food Chart Report

Low Acid Diet

excerpts from **The New York Times**

Tired of Feeling the Burn? *Low-Acid Diet* ***May Help***

Stomach acid has long been blamed for acid reflux, heartburn and other ills. But now some experts are starting to think that the problems may lie not just in the acid coming up from the stomach but in the food going down.

Recent studies have shown a link between bone health and a low-acid diet, while some reports suggest that the acidity of the Western diet increases the risk of diabetes and heart disease.

This year, a small study found that restricting dietary acid could relieve reflux symptoms like coughing and hoarseness in patients who had not been helped by drug therapy, according to the journal Annals of Otology, Rhinology & Laryngology.

Exploring a **Low-Acid Diet** for Bone Health

Why are osteoporotic fractures relatively rare in Asian countries like Japan, where people live as long or longer than Americans and consume almost no calcium-rich dairy products? Why, in Western countries that consume the most dairy foods, are rates of osteoporotic fractures among the highest in the world? And why has no consistent link been found

Alkaline and Acidic Food Chart Report

between the amount of calcium people consume and protection against osteoporosis?

An alternative theory of bone health is the theory of low-acid eating, a diet laden with fruits and vegetables but relatively low in acid-producing protein and moderate in cereal grains.

Studies by Dr. Bess Dawson-Hughes, at the Jean Mayer U.S.D.A. Human Nutrition Research Center on Aging at Tufts University, and collaborators have demonstrated the acid-neutralizing ability of fruits and vegetables and the crucial role they can play in maintaining healthy bones.

Today, there is a general consensus that diet can markedly affect acid-base status and that a person's acid load can be specifically manipulated by dietary means. An established method of estimating acid loads of foods or diets is by calculating the potential renal acid load (PRAL). PRAL provides an estimate of the production of endogenous acid that exceeds the level of alkali produced for given amounts of foods ingested daily. The concept of PRAL calculation is physiologically based and takes into account different intestinal absorption rates of individual minerals and of sulfurcontaining protein, as well as the amount of sulfate produced from metabolized proteins. This method of calculation was experimentally validated in healthy adults, and it showed that, under controlled

Alkaline and Acidic Food Chart Report

conditions, acid loads and renal net acid excretion (NAE) can be reliably estimated from diet composition.

Alkaline Diet Research

Muscle mass gradually declines after age 50, and muscle loss leads to muscle weakness; greater risks of falls, fractures, and disability; and loss of independence. There is plausible evidence that the composition of diets with respect to acid-base balance is a contributing factor.

Protein and cereal grains are metabolized to acidic residues, and fruit and vegetables are metabolized to alkaline residues. In general, American diets are acidic, generating 75–100 mEq acid/d. With the decline in renal function that occurs with aging, older persons are not able to excrete the excess hydrogen ions, and they develop mild but slowly increasing metabolic acidosis. Metabolic acidosis has been linked to muscle wasting in chronic renal failure and in obese subjects who were acidotic while following weight-loss diets; correction of the acidosis has been shown to reverse the muscle wasting in these 2 conditions.

Fruits Low in Acidity

List of fruits lowest in acidity based on PRAL values.

Alkaline and Acidic Food Chart Report

Low-Acid Fruits based on PRAL values	PRAL value
Apricots, dehydrated (low-moisture), sulfured, uncooked	-33
Bananas, dehydrated, or banana powder	-30
Apricots, dried, sulfured, uncooked	-22
Peaches, dehydrated (low-moisture), sulfured, uncooked	-22
Prunes, dehydrated (low-moisture), uncooked	-19
Peaches, dried, sulfured, uncooked	-16
Litchis, dried	-16
Figs, dried, uncooked	-14
Dates, medjool	-14
Raisins, seeded	-14
Fruit, mixed, (prune and apricot and pear), dried	-14
Persimmons, japanese, dried	-14
Currants, zante, dried	-14

Alkaline and Acidic Food Chart Report

Plums, dried (prunes), uncooked	-13
Apricots, dehydrated (low-moisture), sulfured, stewed	-13
Dates, deglet noor	-12
Raisins, seedless	-12
Apples, dehydrated (low moisture), sulfured, uncooked	-12
Orange juice, frozen concentrate, unsweetened, undiluted	-12
Tamarinds, raw	-11
Raisins, golden seedless	-11
Plantains, yellow, fried, Latino restaurant	-10
Breadfruit, raw	-10
Pineapple juice, frozen concentrate, unsweetened, undiluted	-10
Plantains, raw	-10
Pears, dried, sulfured, uncooked	-9
Jackfruit, raw	-9
Grapefruit juice, white, frozen concentrate,	-9

Alkaline and Acidic Food Chart Report

unsweetened, undiluted

Apple juice, frozen concentrate, unsweetened, undiluted, with added ascorbic acid	-9

Low-Acid Fruits based on PRAL values	PRAL value
Apple juice, frozen concentrate, unsweetened, undiluted, without added ascorbic acid	-9
Avocados, raw, California	-9
Peaches, dehydrated (low-moisture), sulfured, stewed	-9
Plantains, green, fried	-9
Plantains, cooked	-9
Tangerine juice, frozen concentrate, sweetened, undiluted	-8
Sapote, mamey, raw	-8
Avocados, raw, all commercial varieties	-8
Apricots, dried, sulfured, stewed, without added sugar	-8
Apples, dried, sulfured, uncooked	-8

Alkaline and Acidic Food Chart Report

Apricots, dried, sulfured, stewed, with added sugar	-8
Jujube, dried	-8
Durian, raw or frozen	-8
Roselle, raw	-7
Custard-apple, (bullock's-heart), raw	-7
Rhubarb, raw	-7
Guavas, common, raw	-7
Bananas, raw	-7
Carissa, (natal-plum), raw	-6
Orange peel, raw	-6
Plums, dried (prunes), stewed, with added sugar	-6
Plums, dried (prunes), stewed, without added sugar	-6
Prunes, dehydrated (low-moisture), stewed	-6
Prickly pears, raw	-6
Figs, dried, stewed	-6
Kiwifruit, gold, raw	-6

Alkaline and Acidic Food Chart Report

Kiwifruit, green, raw	-6
Longans, dried	-6
Guavas, strawberry, raw	-6
Nance, frozen, unsweetened	-6
Passion-fruit juice, purple, raw	-6

Low-Acid Fruits based on PRAL values	PRAL value
Avocados, raw, Florida	-6
Melon balls, frozen	-6
Peaches, dried, sulfured, stewed, with added sugar	-5
Figs, raw	-5
Orange juice, chilled, includes from concentrate, fortified with calcium	-5
Cherimoya, raw	-5
Abiyuch, raw	-5
Currants, european black, raw	-5
Passion-fruit juice, yellow, raw	-5

Alkaline and Acidic Food Chart Report

Prune juice, canned	-5
Peaches, dried, sulfured, stewed, without added sugar	-5
Elderberries, raw	-5
Loquats, raw	-5
Melons, cantaloupe, raw	-5
Soursop, raw	-5
Pears, dried, sulfured, stewed, without added sugar	-5
Nance, canned, syrup, drained	-5
Orange juice, chilled, includes from concentrate, fortified with calcium and vitamin D	-5
Passion-fruit, (granadilla), purple, raw	-5
Rhubarb, frozen, uncooked	-5
Grapes, muscadine, raw	-4
Jujube, raw	-4
Papayas, raw	-4
Grapes, american type (slip skin), raw	-4

Alkaline and Acidic Food Chart Report

Pears, dried, sulfured, stewed, with added sugar	-4
Apricots, frozen, sweetened	-4
Sapodilla, raw	-4
Melons, casaba, raw	-4
Apricots, raw	-4
Oranges, raw, Florida	-4
Currants, red and white, raw	-4

Low-Acid Fruits based on PRAL values	PRAL value
Oranges, raw, all commercial varieties	-4
Longans, raw	-4
Melons, honeydew, raw	-4
Lemon peel, raw	-4
Sugar-apples, (sweetsop), raw	-4
Guava sauce, cooked	-4
Kumquats, raw	-4

Alkaline and Acidic Food Chart Report

Pomegranate juice, bottled	-4
Rhubarb, frozen, cooked, with sugar	-4
Oranges, raw, with peel	-4
Orange juice, raw	-4
Cherries, sweet, raw	-4
Quinces, raw	-4
Pummelo, raw	-4
Prunes, canned, heavy syrup pack, solids and liquids	-4
Naranjilla (lulo) pulp, frozen, unsweetened	-4
Crabapples, raw	-4

Printed in Great Britain
by Amazon